Table of Contents

Introduction

Are you struggling with your weight or health issues like diabetes, chronic fatigue, or inflammation? These problems nearly always link back to diet and improper nutrition. What we eat has a huge impact on every aspect of our bodies and minds, and when we aren't careful, we end up consuming food that actively hurts our health.

Switching to the Vegetarian Keto diet could change your life and improve your health for the long-term. What this diet does is restrict the amount of carbs you eat and replace them with healthy fats found in food like avocados, nuts, and seeds. The body then becomes to burn fat for energy, resulting in benefits like weight loss and sharper cognitive abilities. Benefits can increase when you combine the Keto diet with vegetarianism, so your protein and fat comes from plant sources, eggs, and full-fat dairy.

The next few chapters introduce you to the Vegetarian Keto diet in more detail, so you understand the science behind it and the health benefits that follow. You'll learn what you can and can't eat, as well as do's and don'ts that make the diet easier to follow. The right food can change your life for the better, and in 30 days, you'll be a true believer.

Chapter 1: What Is The Vegetarian Keto Diet?

The Vegetarian Keto diet combines the traditional vegetarian diet with the Ketogenic diet. You're most likely familiar with vegetarianism, but what is the Keto diet exactly? The goal of this eating lifestyle is to eliminate a significant number of carbs and replace them with healthy fat. Normally, the body resorts to carbs for energy, but when fat makes up 60-75% of your daily calories, the body begins to produce ketones and burn fat for fuel instead.

On the traditional Keto diet, you get the fats and protein you need from meat, but when you add vegetarianism into the mix, it looks quite different. It can be challenging to get into ketosis on a plant-based diet because most vegetarians eat more carbs and less fat than meat-eaters. The solution is to emphasis vegetable fats and oils, such as:

Avocados - An excellent source of monounsaturated fat and vitamins, as well as fiber.

Macadamia nuts - This type of nut is one of the best nut sources for fat.

Pumpkin seeds - A great snack, this seed is high in fat and low in carbs with a good amount of protein.

Coconut oil - A great source of saturated fat and medium-chain triglycerides, which the body transforms easily into ketones.

What about eggs and dairy?

The Keto diet includes eggs and full-fat dairy, and while some vegetarians eliminate one or both from their diet, we can't recommend you do that. That resembles a vegan diet, which is very difficult when combined with trying to get into ketosis. Eggs will be a very important source of protein and fat, while full-fat dairy contains nutrients like calcium, short-chain fatty acids, and more.

The Vegetarian Ketogenic Diet In A Nutshell

To follow the Vegetarian Keto diet faithfully, here's a summary of what you have to do:

Cut out all meat, fish, and poultry

Eat only 20-35 grams of carbs per day

Have fat compose 70% of your daily calories

Have protein compose 25% of your daily calories

Eat lots of low-carb vegetables high in nutrients

If necessary, take supplements like iron and zinc to fill in gaps from not eating meat

Chapter 2: Benefits Of The Vegetarian Keto Diet

There are good reasons to be vegetarian and good reasons to be on the Keto diet. When you combine the diets, you end up enjoying both sets of benefits. The Keto diet even counters some of the issues with vegetarianism, like consuming too many carbs, processed foods, and sugar. Let's explore the most significant pros of the Vegetarian Keto diet:

Easier weight loss

Carbs - not fat - are the reason why so many people are overweight. When the body uses carbs as fuel, a lot of the resulting glucose ends up being stored as body fat. When you cut out those carbs, the body is forced to burn fat instead of store it, resulting in easier weight loss.

Weight loss is still about burning more calories than you eat, which is where the vegetarian aspect of the diet comes in handy. Plant protein is much lower in calories than meat protein, so it's easier to avoid overeating. Additionally, many of the carbs found in vegetables are fiber carbs, which don't count towards your daily carb intake. You can eat more vegetables than meat, get the nutrients and satisfaction you need from your food, and burn fat - the pounds slip away much more effectively.

Brain protection

Your brain loves healthy fat, which makes sense considering it's mostly made of fat (plus water). Sticking to the Vegetarian Keto diet gives your brain the fuel it craves and protects it from all kinds of neurodegenerative conditions like Alzheimer's. As for more immediate benefits, eliminating refined carbs from your diet also clears up what's known as "brain fog," which is possibly caused by inflammation. Sugar and other junk food aggravate the entire body, resulting in said inflammation, so avoiding those out gives your body and brain the healing time it needs. Vegetarian-Keto foods like berries, seeds, and nuts do their part to encourage brain's balance of chemicals, so it works more effectively.

Protection against disease

In addition to Alzheimer's, a Vegetarian Keto diet protects you against other diseases like diabetes. Unlike carbs, fat doesn't affect your blood sugar, so your insulin levels stay balanced. If you have type 2 diabetes, being in ketosis can even help significantly reduce your symptoms.

The diet can also protect you against heart disease and other metabolic syndromes like high blood pressure, high blood sugar, and low HDL cholesterol. The Vegetarian Keto diet is full of heart-healthy foods like berries, dark leafy greens, pumpkin seeds, and Greek yogurt.

More energy

A diet high in carbs, especially refined ones, results in a heavy, tired feeling. It's also common to feel a surge of energy after eating, but then the crash follows. This happens with all carbs, not just sugar. Switching to fat for fuel means you're eating foods known for their energy-boosting qualities, and the carbs you do eat from vegetables are slow-burning. Your energy levels are more balanced, so you don't experience that surge-'n-crash.

Not eating meat brings its own energy benefits. Plants are full of fiber, which keeps your body cleared out. You can eat a giant plate of vegetables and feel light and energetic, while if you ate just half of that amount in meat, odds are you'll want a nap.

Chapter 3: What You Can And Can't Eat

You know what the Vegetarian Keto diet is and why it's so good for you, so let's go over what the diet actually looks like in practice. Your food list consists of plant protein sources, lots of vegetables, some fruit, dairy, seeds and nuts, and oils. The list of foods you *can't* eat include all grains, all refined sugars, high-carb vegetables and fruit, and any kind of processed food.

Here's what you *can* eat:

Protein

Tempeh

Tofu

Seitan

Eggs

Vegetables

Dark leafy vegetables (spinach, kale, collard greens, etc)

Broccoli

Cauliflower

Zucchini

Asparagus

Green beans

Bell peppers

Tomatoes

Mushrooms

Onions

Cabbage

Garlic

Fruit

Avocadoes

Raspberries

Blackberries

Blackberries

Lemons

Limes

Full-fat dairy

Hard cheeses

Mozzarella

Brie

Muenster

Monterey jack

Heavy cream

Butter

Ghee

Greek yogurt

Cottage cheese

Sour cream

Cream cheese

Nuts/seeds

Almonds (in moderation)

Walnuts (in moderation)

Hazelnuts (in moderation)

Macadamia nuts

Brazil nuts

Pecans

Pumpkin seeds

Sunflower seeds

Flax seeds

Chia seeds

Fats/oils

Coconut oil

MCT oil

Extra virgin olive oil

Natural (or homemade) no-sugar added nut butters

Sweeteners

Stevia

Erythritol

Monk fruit

Allulose

Condiments/baking supplies

Hot sauce

Soy sauce

Yellow mustard

Sugar-free ketchup

Sugar-free sauerkraut

Sugar-free, high-fat salad dressings

Coconut flour

Almond flour

Arrowroot powder

Baking powder

Baking soda

Natural flavor extracts (like sugar-free vanilla)

Beverages

Unsweetened coconut water

Unsweetened nut milks

Herbal teas

Black coffee

Here's what you *cannot* eat:

<u>Grains</u>

Wheat

Corn

White rice

Wild rice

Cornmeal

Cereals

Oatmeal

Quinoa

Buckwheat

Barley

Spelt

<u>High-glycemic vegetables</u>

Carrots

Potatoes

Yams

Parsnips

Beets

Pumpkins

Dairy

Cow's milk

Low-low/no-fat dairy products

Legumes

Lentils

Green peas

Black beans

Kidney beans

White beans

High-glycemic fruit

Apples

Bananas

Grapes

Strawberries

Apricots

Pears

Plums

All dried fruit

Pineapple

Watermelon

Sweeteners

Honey

Agave

Maple syrup

White sugar

Brown dark

Molasses

Chapter 4: Do's And Don'ts Of The Vegetarian Keto Diet

The Vegetarian Keto diet is challenging and restrictive because you're cutting out entire food groups (grains and meat). If you get stuck on every little detail, it can get overwhelming and won't work for the long-term. There are a handful of "do's and don'ts" you can remember that keep you looking at the big picture. Here are the most helpful four "do's" and three "don'ts:"

Do: Eat real food

The most important part of the Vegetarian Keto diet is eating *real* food. Anything that's been overly-processed or packed with additives is off the table, even if it claims to be Keto or vegetarian-friendly. If you're getting something in a package or can, you want it to have as few ingredients as possible. All those ingredients should be natural

Do: Remember your electrolytes

When you eliminate processed foods from your diet, you'll find you're getting significantly less sodium. Remember to use a good Himalayan salt for your food. Another way to get electrolytes is to drink bone broth (preferably homemade with salt), which has additional benefits. If you begin experiencing what's known as the "Keto flu," salted bone broth can help relieve the headaches, fatigue, and hunger pangs.

Do: Use natural zero-calorie sweeteners

Not eating sugar can be really difficult for a lot of people. We're used to sugary foods; even store-bought bread is full of it. To make food taste more "normal" to you, use natural sweeteners that are zero-calorie. These won't add to your carb intake and don't come with the issues that artificial zero-cal sweeteners do. Use stevia, monk fruit, and blends in your coffee, tea, and homemade Keto-approved baked goods.

Do: Eat iron-rich foods and Vitamin C together

One of the concerns about the vegetarian aspect of this diet is that you don't get enough iron. The iron in plants isn't as easily-digested as the iron in meat products, but when you eat plant iron alongside vitamin C, it helps the body absorb it. Load up on food like spinach, tofu, sunflower seeds, and spirulina. Spinach and spirulina contain *both* iron and calcium, so they're a really good choice. Keep in that mind that tea and coffee can hinder iron absorption, so cut back if you need to. Too much calcium can also impact the body's ability to absorb iron, so be aware of that. Talk to your doctor before considering iron and/or vitamin C supplements.

Don't: Ignore your protein intake

The Vegetarian Keto diet isn't a high-protein diet, but protein is still very important, especially if you're hoping to lose weight. On the traditional Keto diet, getting enough protein is rarely a problem, but when you eliminate meat, it might be trickier. Make sure every meal contains a good plant protein and consider using a plant-based protein powder like Vega Essentials or Sun Warrior.

Don't: Get hung up on your ketone levels

When you get started on the Vegetarian Keto diet, you'll want to measure your ketone levels using either a urine, blood, or breath test. Ketosis occurs anywhere between 0.5-3.0 mmol/L. Some people get really focused on getting their ketone levels really high, but that can be dangerous since ketones make the blood acidic. Also, benefits don't improve above 3.0 mmol/L, and if you have diabetes, you don't want to be higher than 0.5.

Don't obsess over checking your ketones all the time; pay more attention to how you're feeling. After a while, your tests won't even show that your ketone levels are up, because your body is using them.

Don't: Go crazy on the cheese

People get excited that they can eat cheese on the Vegetarian Keto diet, but you want to watch how much you're eating. Cheese is by no means a "health food," and it's high in calories and saturated fat, which isn't the best fat for your body. The lactose can also bother your stomach if you eat too much. Various hard and soft cheeses can be a valuable part of your meal plans, but don't depend on it to be the star of every dish or snack.

30 Days Ketogenic Vegetarian Meal Plan, Top 90 Ketogenic Vegetarian Recipes

DAY 1

1-Delicious Strawberry Muffins

Time: 25 minutes

Serve: 12

Ingredients:

- 2/3 cup fresh strawberries, diced
- 3 eggs
- 1 tsp ground cinnamon
- 2 tsp baking powder
- 2 1/2 cups almond flour
- 1/3 cup heavy cream
- 1 tsp vanilla
- 1/2 cup Swerve
- 5 tbsp butter

Directions:

- Preheat the oven to 350 F/ 176 C.
- Spray muffin tray with cooking spray and set aside.
- Add butter and sweetener in a bowl and beat together using a hand blender until smooth.
- Add eggs, cream, and vanilla and beat until frothy.
- In another bowl, sift together almond flour, cinnamon, baking powder, and salt.
- Add almond flour mixture to wet ingredients and mix until well combined.
- Add strawberries and stir well.
- Pour batter into the prepared muffin tray and bake in preheated oven for 15-20 minutes.
- Serve and enjoy.

Nutritional Value (Amount per Serving):

- Calories 208
- Fat 18.8 g
- Carbohydrates 6.4 g
- Sugar 1.3 g
- Protein 6.6 g
- Cholesterol 58 mg

Flavorful Caprese Salad

Time: 15 minutes

Serve: 4

Ingredients:

- 4 cups spinach
- 1/4 cup basil, chopped
- 1/2 cup cherry tomatoes, halved
- 1 avocado, chopped
- 1 cup mozzarella balls, halved
- 1 cup strawberries, quartered
- Pepper
- Salt
- For dressing:
- 1/2 tsp dried oregano
- 2 garlic cloves, minced
- 1 1/2 tbsp balsamic vinegar
- 2 tbsp red wine vinegar
- 3 tbsp mayonnaise
- 3 tbsp olive oil
- Pepper
- Salt

Directions:

- In a large mixing bowl, toss together avocado, basil, mozzarella, strawberries, and tomatoes.
- Divide spinach between four serving plates and top with caprese mixture.
- In a small bowl, combine together all dressing ingredients.
- Drizzle dressing over salad and serve.

Nutritional Value (Amount per Serving):

- Calories 283
- Fat 25.6 g
- Carbohydrates 12.7 g
- Sugar 3.5 g
- Protein 4.5 g
- Cholesterol 7 mg

Broccoli Cauliflower Risotto

Time: 25 minutes

Serve: 2

Ingredients:

- 1 broccoli head, cut into florets
- 1 cauliflower head, cut into florets
- 1 tbsp lemon zest
- 1/2 cup vegetable stock
- 2 tbsp butter
- 2 onion spring, chopped
- 1/2 cup parmesan cheese, grated
- 2 tbsp cream
- 1/2 tsp pepper
- 1/2 tsp salt

Directions:

- Add cauliflower and broccoli florets into the food processor and process until it looks like rice.
- Melt butter in a large saucepan over medium heat.
- Add onion and sauté for 2 minutes.
- Add broccoli and cauliflower rice and sauté for 2-3 minutes.
- Add stock and cover and cook for 10 minutes. Stir occasionally.
- Add parmesan cheese and cream. Season with lemon zest. Stir until cheese is melted.
- Serve and enjoy.

Nutritional Value (Amount per Serving):

- Calories 314
- Fat 22.1 g
- Carbohydrates 11.9 g
- Sugar 4.9 g
- Protein 16.7 g
- Cholesterol 63 mg

DAY 2

2-Yummy Pecan Muffins

Time: 30 minutes

Serve: 12

Ingredients:

- 4 eggs
- 1/2 cup pecans, chopped
- 1/2 tsp ground cinnamon
- 2 tsp allspice
- 1 tsp vanilla
- 1/4 cup almond milk
- 2 tbsp butter, melted
- 1/2 cup swerve sweetener
- 1 tsp psyllium husk
- 1 tbsp baking powder
- 1 1/2 cups almond flour

Directions:

- Preheat the oven to 400 F/ 204 C.
- Spray muffin tray with cooking spray and set aside.
- Beat eggs, almond milk, vanilla, sweetener, and butter in a bowl using a hand blender until smooth.
- Add remaining ingredients and mix until well combined.
- Pour batter into the prepared muffin tray and bake in preheated oven for 15-20 minutes.
- Serve and enjoy.

Nutritional Value (Amount per Serving):

- Calories 205
- Fat 18.6 g
- Carbohydrates 6.7 g
- Sugar 1.2 g
- Protein 6 g
- Cholesterol 60 mg

Cheesy Cauliflower Fritter

Time: 30 minutes

Serve: 4

Ingredients:

- 2 large eggs
- 1 jalapeno, sliced
- 1 tbsp coconut flour
- 3/4 cup almond flour
- 1/4 cup Mexican cheese, shredded
- 3 cups cauliflower florets
- 1/4 tsp salt

Directions:

- Add cauliflower florets into the pot of boiling water and boil until cauliflower is softened. Drain the water.
- Heat pan over medium-low heat. Lightly spray with cooking spray.
- Add boiled cauliflower in a blender with remaining ingredients and blend until smooth.
- Scoop 1/4 cup of batter and place on the pan to form one fritter. Cook for 5 minutes then flip and cook for 3-5 minutes more until both sides are lightly browned.
- Serve and enjoy.

Nutritional Value (Amount per Serving):

- Calories 301
- Fat 22.6 g
- Carbohydrates 11.9 g
- Sugar 3.1 g
- Protein 16.7 g
- Cholesterol 123 mg

Creamy Parmesan Broccoli Soup

Time: 40 minutes

Serve: 2

Ingredients:

- 1 broccoli head, cut into florets
- 1/2 cup parmesan cheese, grated
- 3 cups vegetable stock
- 1 lemon juice
- 2 garlic cloves, chopped
- 2 tbsp olive oil
- 1/2 tsp pepper
- 1/2 tsp salt

Directions:

- Heat oil in a saucepan over medium heat.
- Add garlic and sauté for 3 minutes.
- Add broccoli and sauté for 5 minutes.
- Add stock, bring to boil, cover and simmer for 20 minutes.
- Remove saucepan from heat and using blender puree the soup until smooth and creamy.
- Add parmesan cheese and lemon juice and blend until smooth.
- Serve and enjoy.

Nutritional Value (Amount per Serving):

- Calories 323
- Fat 28.2 g
- Carbohydrates 8.7 g
- Sugar 3.8 g
- Protein 17.1 g
- Cholesterol 29 mg

DAY 3

Fluffy Breakfast Waffles

Time: 20 minutes

Serve: 4

Ingredients:

- 2 eggs
- 1 1/4 cup almond milk
- 2 tbsp butter, melted
- 2 tbsp swerve
- 1 tbsp maple extract
- 1 tsp baking soda
- 1/2 tsp baking powder
- 2 tbsp coconut flour
- 1 1/2 cups almond flour

Directions:

- Add all ingredients to a large mixing bowl and mix until well combined. Let sit for 5 minutes.
- Preheat the waffle iron and coat with cooking spray.
- Pour prepared batter into preheated waffle iron and cook for 3-4 minutes or until lightly golden brown on each side.
- Serve and enjoy.

Nutritional Value (Amount per Serving):

- Calories 345
- Fat 32 g
- Carbohydrates 10.5 g
- Protein 7.6 g
- Cholesterol 97 mg

Thai Zoodles

Time: 10 minutes

Serve: 4

Ingredients:

- 1 egg
- 2 medium zucchini, spiralized
- 3 tbsp scallions, chopped
- 3 tbsp nuts, chopped
- 1/2 onion, chopped
- 2 tbsp olive oil
- 1/2 lime juice
- 1 garlic clove, minced
- 2 tbsp coconut sugar
- 1 tsp chili sauce
- 1 tbsp coconut aminos
- 3 tbsp unsweetened almond butter
- 2.50 oz water

Directions:

- Whisk together water, lime juice, garlic, coconut sugar, chili sauce, coconut aminos, and almond butter in a bowl and set aside.
- In a medium pan, heat oil and sauté the chopped onion until softened.
- Add egg in onion and stir gently about 1 minute to cook the eggs and break them up into small pieces.
- Stir in spiralized zucchini noodles and sauce and cook for few minutes.
- Add chopped scallions and nuts and cook for another minute.
- Serve immediately and enjoy.

Nutritional Value (Amount per Serving):

- Calories 116
- Fat 6.9 g
- Carbohydrates 12 g
- Sugar 8.7 g
- Protein 3.9 g
- Cholesterol 41 mg

Roasted Cauliflower

Time: 1 hour 25 minutes

Serve: 2

Ingredients:

- 1 whole cauliflower head, trim outer leaves
- 1/4 cup parmesan cheese, grated
- 2 tbsp olive oil
- 1 tsp garlic powder
- 1 lemon juice
- 4 tbsp butter, melted
- 3 tbsp Dijon mustard
- 1/2 tsp pepper
- 1/2 tsp salt

Directions:

- Preheat the oven to 425 F/ 220 C.
- Place cauliflower on a baking dish.
- In a small bowl, mix together butter, oil, lemon juice, mustard, garlic powder, pepper, and salt.
- Brush cauliflower with butter mixture and bake in preheated oven for an hour or until tender.
- Remove from oven and sprinkle with parmesan cheese. Return to the oven and cook for 5-8 minutes or until cheese melted.
- Serve and enjoy.

Nutritional Value (Amount per Serving):

- Calories 658
- Fat 56 g
- Carbohydrates 5.1 g
- Sugar 1.6 g
- Protein 26.6 g
- Cholesterol 121 mg

DAY 4

Low-Carb Keto Oatmeal

Time: 30 minutes

Serve: 1

Ingredients:

- 1 tbsp erythritol
- 1 tbsp coconut oil
- 1 tsp ground cinnamon
- 1 tbsp coconut flakes
- 1 tbsp chia seeds
- 1 tbsp flax meal
- 1/2 cup hemp hearts
- 1 cup unsweetened coconut milk

Directions:

- Add all ingredients into the small saucepan and stir to combine.
- Bring to simmer over medium heat until thickened. Stir occasionally.
- Serve and enjoy.

Nutritional Value (Amount per Serving):

- Calories 192
- Fat 18 g
- Carbohydrates 14 g
- Sugar 8.7 g
- Protein 4.2 g
- Cholesterol 1 mg

Mexican Salad

Time: 15 minutes

Serve: 4

Ingredients:

- 1 small tomato, diced
- 1 avocado, diced
- 1/4 cup cheddar cheese, shredded
- 1/2 lemon juice
- 1/4 cup mayonnaise
- 1/2 cup salsa
- 1 bag frozen cauliflower
- 1 tbsp cilantro, chopped
- 1 tsp onion powder
- 1 tsp chili powder
- 1 tsp paprika
- 1 tsp cumin
- Pepper
- Salt

Directions:

- Add cauliflower in a microwave-safe dish and microwave on high for 4 minutes or until tender.
- Mix together salsa, seasonings, lemon juice, and mayonnaise.
- Stir in cauliflower. Fold in cheese, tomato, herbs, and avocado.
- Place in refrigerator for 2 hours.
- Serve and enjoy.

Nutritional Value (Amount per Serving):

- Calories 149
- Fat 9 g
- Carbohydrates 14 g
- Sugar 5.6 g
- Protein 5.4 g
- Cholesterol 11 mg

Spicy Cauliflower Zucchini Rice

Time: 35 minutes

Serve: 2

Ingredients:

- 1 cauliflower head, cut into florets
- 1/2 tsp paprika
- 1/2 tsp garlic powder
- 1/2 tsp cayenne pepper
- 1/2 tsp cumin
- 1/2 tsp chili powder
- 6 onion spring, chopped
- 2 jalapenos, chopped
- 4 tbsp olive oil
- 1 zucchini, trimmed and cut into cubes
- 1/2 tsp black pepper
- 1/2 tsp salt

Directions:

- Preheat the oven to 400 F/ 200 C.
- Add cauliflower florets into the food processor and process until it looks like rice.
- Transfer cauliflower rice to a baking tray and drizzle with half oil.
- Bake in preheated oven for 15 minutes, turn halfway through.
- Heat remaining oil in a pan over medium heat.
- Add zucchini and cook for 5-8 minutes.
- Add onion and jalapenos and cook for 5 minutes.
- Add spices and stir well. Set aside.
- Add cauliflower rice in zucchini mixture and stir until well coated.
- Serve and enjoy.

Nutritional Value (Amount per Serving):

- Calories 255
- Fat 28.7 g
- Carbohydrates 12.3 g
- Sugar 5.2 g
- Protein 4.3 g
- Cholesterol 0 mg

DAY 5

Healthy Green Smoothie

Time: 10 minutes

Serve: 1

Ingredients:

- 1 tbsp swerve
- 2 tbsp almond butter
- 1 tsp chia seeds
- 1/2 cup spinach
- 3 strawberries

Directions:

- Add all ingredients to the blender and blend until smooth and creamy.
- Serve immediately and enjoy.

Nutritional Value (Amount per Serving):

- Calories 245
- Fat 19 g
- Carbohydrates 11 g
- Sugar 2.6 g
- Protein 8 g
- Cholesterol 0 mg

Parmesan Zucchini Pizza

Time: 20 minutes

Serve: 4

Ingredients:

- 1 egg
- 1/2 packet ranch seasoning mix
- 1/4 cup parmesan cheese, grated
- 2 cups zucchini, shredded

Directions:

- Preheat the oven to 450 F/ 232 C.
- Combine together zucchini, parmesan cheese, seasoning, and egg in a bowl and mix well.
- Spray pizza pan with cooking spray and press zucchini mixture onto the pan evenly into a circle about half inch thick.
- Bake pizza in preheated oven for 15 minutes.
- Serve and enjoy.

Nutritional Value (Amount per Serving):

- Calories 265
- Fat 17.2 g
- Carbohydrates 6 g
- Sugar 1.1 g
- Protein 26.1 g
- Cholesterol 101 mg

Cheese Broccoli Stuffed Peppers

Time: 1 hour 10 minutes

Serve: 2

Ingredients:

- 4 eggs
- 1/2 cup cheddar cheese, grated
- 1/2 tsp garlic powder
- 1 tsp dried thyme
- 1/4 cup feta cheese, crumbled
- 1/2 cup broccoli, cooked
- 2 bell peppers, cut in half and remove seeds
- 1/4 tsp pepper
- 1/2 tsp salt

Directions:

- Preheat the oven to 350 F/ 180 C.
- Place bell peppers half in a baking dish. Cut side up.
- Stuff feta and broccoli into the peppers.
- Beat egg in a bowl with seasoning and pour egg mixture into the pepper cases over feta and broccoli.
- Bake in preheated oven for 45-50 minutes.
- Add grated cheese on top and bake for 10 minutes more or until cheese melted.
- Serve and enjoy.

Nutritional Value (Amount per Serving):

- Calories 339
- Fat 22.5 g
- Carbohydrates 13.3 g
- Sugar 8.2 g
- Protein 22.8 g
- Cholesterol 374 mg

DAY 6

Super Easy Pancake

Time: 15 minutes

Serve: 1

Ingredients:

- 2 large eggs
- 1 tsp lemon zest
- 1 tsp swerve
- 2 tbsp almond flour
- 2 oz cream cheese

Directions:

- Heat pan over medium heat and spray with cooking spray.
- Add all ingredients to the blender and blend until mixed.
- Pour batter into a hot pan and make small pancakes.
- Cook pancakes from both the sides until lightly golden brown.
- Serve and enjoy.

Nutritional Value (Amount per Serving):

- Calories 427
- Fat 36.7 g
- Carbohydrates 7.7 g
- Sugar 1.5 g
- Protein 19.9 g
- Cholesterol 434 mg

Delicious Jalapeno Pizza

Time: 25 minutes

Serve: 4

Ingredients:

- 1 cup cheddar cheese, shredded
- 2 jalapeno pepper, sliced
- 1/3 cup almond flour
- 1/4 tsp garlic powder
- 1 egg, beaten
- 3/4 cup mozzarella cheese, shredded
- 2 oz cream cheese

Directions:

- Preheat the oven to 350 F/ 176 C.
- In a small bowl, add mozzarella cheese and cream cheese. Microwave on high for 20 seconds or until melted.
- Add remaining ingredients to the melted cheese and mix well.
- Spray 10-inch pan with cooking spray and spread the dough out evenly.
- Bake in preheated oven for 10 minutes. Top with jalapenos and cheese and continue for another 10 minutes.
- Serve and enjoy.

Nutritional Value (Amount per Serving):

- Calories 250
- Fat 21 g
- Carbohydrates 3.6 g
- Sugar 0.9 g
- Protein 13.1 g
- Cholesterol 89 mg

Creamy Cabbage

Time: 25 minutes

Serve: 4

Ingredients:

- 3 oz cream cheese
- 1/2 cabbage head, shredded
- 2 garlic cloves, chopped
- 1 onion, sliced
- 1 bell pepper, cut into strips
- 2 tbsp butter
- 1/2 tsp pepper
- 1 tsp kosher salt

Directions:

- Melt butter in a saucepan over medium heat.
- Add garlic and onion and sauté for 5 minutes.
- Add cabbage and bell pepper and cook for 5-8 minutes or until softened.
- Add cream cheese and stir well.
- Season with pepper and salt.
- Serve and enjoy.

Nutritional Value (Amount per Serving):

- Calories 171
- Fat 13.4 g
- Carbohydrates 11.2 g
- Sugar 5.6 g
- Protein 3.5 g
- Cholesterol 39 mg

DAY 7

Yummy Mug Cake

Time: 10 minutes

Serve: 1

Ingredients:

- 1 egg, beaten
- 1 tbsp sugar-free chocolate chips
- 1/2 tsp baking powder
- 1 tbsp cocoa powder
- 2 tbsp swerve
- 1 tbsp coconut flour
- 1 tbsp butter, melted

Directions:

- Add all ingredients into the microwave safe coffee mug and mix well.
- Place in microwave and microwave on high for 60 seconds.
- Serve and enjoy.

Nutritional Value (Amount per Serving):

- Calories 216
- Fat 18 g
- Carbohydrates 7.5 g
- Sugar 1.5 g
- Protein 8.5 g
- Cholesterol 194 mg

Tasty Tomato Soup

Time: 45 minutes

Serve: 6

Ingredients:

- 10 medium tomato, cut into cubes
- 2 tbsp fresh basil, minced
- 1/4 cup heavy cream
- 1/4 cup water
- 4 garlic cloves, minced
- 1 tbsp olive oil
- 1/4 tsp pepper
- 1/2 tsp sea salt

Directions:

- Preheat the oven to 400 F/ 204 C.
- Spray a baking tray with cooking spray and set aside.
- In a bowl, toss together tomato, garlic, and olive oil.
- Spread tomato onto a baking tray and roast in preheated oven for 20-25 minutes/
- Transfer tomato into a blender and blend until smooth.
- Pour tomato puree into a small saucepan over medium heat.
- Add water and season with pepper and salt. Simmer for 10-15 minutes.
- Stir in basil and cream.
- Serve and enjoy.

Nutritional Value (Amount per Serving):

- Calories 78
- Fat 4.6 g
- Carbohydrates 8.9 g
- Sugar 5.4 g
- Protein 2.1 g
- Cholesterol 7 mg

Delicious Baked Cauliflower

Time: 55 minutes

Serve: 2

Ingredients:

- 1/2 cauliflower head, cut into florets
- 2 tbsp olive oil
- For seasoning:
- 1/4 tsp dried oregano
- 1/4 tsp dried basil
- 1/4 tsp dried thyme
- 1/2 tsp garlic powder
- 1/2 tsp ground cumin
- 1/2 tsp black pepper
- 1/2 tsp white pepper
- 1 tsp onion powder
- 1 tbsp ground cayenne pepper
- 2 tbsp ground paprika
- 2 tsp salt

Directions:

- Preheat the oven to 400 F/ 200 C.
- Line baking tray with parchment paper and set aside.
- In a large bowl, mix together all seasoning ingredients.
- Add oil and stir well. Add cauliflower to the bowl seasoning mixture and stir well to coat.
- Spread the cauliflower florets over the baking tray and bake in preheated oven for 45 minutes.
- Serve and enjoy.

Nutritional Value (Amount per Serving):

- Calories 177
- Fat 15.6 g
- Carbohydrates 11.5 g
- Sugar 3.2 g
- Protein 3.1 g
- Cholesterol 0 mg

DAY 8

Moist Breakfast Cake

Time: 2 hours

Serve: 12

Ingredients:

- 2 1/2 cups almond flour
- 5 eggs, separated
- 16 drops liquid stevia
- 4 cardamom pods, crushed
- 1 tsp vanilla extract
- 2 tsp orange extract
- 1 tsp baking powder
- 2 oranges, un-waxed and washed

Directions:

- Preheat the oven to 350 F/ 180 C.
- Line Bread tin with parchment paper and set aside.
- Add oranges into a pot filled with water and cover with lid. Bring to boil and simmer for 1 hour.
- Drain the water and let the oranges cool. Cut oranges in half and remove seeds then puree in a blender.
- In a bowl, whisk egg whites until stiff peaks form.
- Add all ingredients except egg whites to the orange pulp and mix well. Fold egg whites until well combined.
- Pour batter into the prepared bread tin and bake in preheated oven for 50 minutes.
- Cut into slices and serve.

Nutritional Value (Amount per Serving):

- Calories 177
- Fat 13.5 g
- Carbohydrates 9.1 g
- Sugar 4 g
- Protein 7.6 g
- Cholesterol 68 mg

Cauliflower Broccoli Salad

Time: 20 minutes

Serve: 7

Ingredients:

- 8 oz cauliflower florets
- 8 oz broccoli florets
- 2 tbsp green onion, chopped
- 4 oz cheddar cheese, cubed
- 2 oz red bell pepper, diced
- For dressing:
- 1 tbsp fresh lemon juice
- 2 tbsp swerve
- 3/4 cup sour cream
- 3/4 cup mayonnaise

Directions:

- Add all salad ingredients to the mixing bowl and toss well.
- In a small bowl, mix together all dressing ingredients and pour over salad.
- Toss well and place in refrigerator for 1-2 hours.
- Serve chilled and enjoy.

Nutritional Value (Amount per Serving):

- Calories 249
- Fat 19.2 g
- Carbohydrates 14 g
- Sugar 4.9 g
- Protein 7 g
- Cholesterol 34 mg

Parmesan Broccoli

Time: 35 minutes

Serve: 2

Ingredients:

- 4 cups broccoli florets
- 1 lemon juice
- 1 cup parmesan cheese, grated
- 4 garlic cloves, sliced
- 3 tbsp coconut oil
- 1/2 tsp pepper
- 1 1/2 tsp salt

Directions:

- Preheat the oven to 425 F/ 220 C.
- In a bowl, toss broccoli florets with coconut oil. Add garlic and season with pepper and salt.
- Spread broccoli on a baking tray and roast in preheated oven for 20 minutes.
- Remove broccoli from the oven and sprinkle with half parmesan cheese and bake for 5 minutes more.
- Add remaining parmesan cheese and lemon juice. Stir well.
- Serve and enjoy.

Nutritional Value (Amount per Serving):

- Calories 548
- Fat 39 g
- Carbohydrates 14 g
- Sugar 3.2 g
- Protein 29.6 g
- Cholesterol 60 mg

DAY 9

Vanilla Donuts

Time: 20 minutes

Serve: 14

Ingredients:

- 4 eggs
- 1 tsp vanilla extract
- 1 tsp baking powder
- 2 tbsp heavy cream
- 1/4 cup Swerve
- 1/3 cup butter, melted
- 1 cup almond flour

Directions:

- Preheat the oven to 350 F/ 175 C.
- Add butter, sweetener, and cream in a food processor and blend until smooth.
- Add vanilla extract and eggs and blend until combined.
- Add almond flour and baking powder and mix well.
- Spoon the batter into greased donut pan and bake in preheated oven for 15 minutes.
- Serve and enjoy.

Nutritional Value (Amount per Serving):

- Calories 111
- Fat 10.4 g
- Carbohydrates 2.1 g
- Sugar 0.4 g
- Protein 3.4 g
- Cholesterol 61 mg

Fresh Asparagus Tomato Salad

Time: 20 minutes

Serve: 4

Ingredients:

- 1/2 lb asparagus, trimmed and cut into pieces
- 8 oz cherry tomatoes, halved
- For dressing:
- 1/4 tsp garlic and herb seasoning blend
- 1 tbsp water
- 2 tbsp olive oil
- 1 tbsp vinegar
- 1 tbsp shallot, minced
- 1 garlic clove, minced

Directions:

- Add 1 tablespoon of water and asparagus in a microwave-safe bowl and cover with cling film and microwave for 2 minutes.
- Remove asparagus from bowl and place into a ice water until cool.
- Add asparagus and tomatoes into a medium bowl.
- In a small bowl, mix together all remaining ingredients and pour over vegetables.
- Toss vegetables well and serve.

Nutritional Value (Amount per Serving):

- Calories 85
- Fat 7.2 g
- Carbohydrates 5.1 g
- Sugar 2.6 g
- Protein 1.9 g
- Cholesterol 0 mg

Delicious Tomato Cauliflower Rice

Time: 25 minutes

Serve: 3

Ingredients:

- 1 cauliflower head, cut into florets
- 2 tbsp olive oil
- 1 tsp white pepper
- 1 tsp black pepper
- 1 tbsp dried thyme
- 2 chilies, chopped
- 2 garlic cloves, chopped
- 1 tomato, chopped
- 1 onion, chopped
- 2 tbsp tomato paste
- 1/2 tsp salt

Directions:

- Preheat the oven to 400 F/ 200 C.
- Add cauliflower florets into the food processor and process until it looks like rice.
- Stir in tomato paste, tomatoes, and spices and mix well.
- Spread cauliflower mixture on a baking tray and drizzle with olive oil.
- Bake in preheated oven for 15 minutes.
- Serve and enjoy.

Nutritional Value (Amount per Serving):

- Calories 138
- Fat 9.7 g
- Carbohydrates 13 g
- Sugar 5.6 g
- Protein 3.2 g
- Cholesterol 0 mg

DAY 10

Grain Free Crepes

Time: 10 minutes

Serve: 6

Ingredients:

- 4 eggs
- 4 tbsp cream cheese
- 2 tbsp psyllium husk
- 4 egg whites
- 2 tbsp butter

Directions:

- Add all ingredients except butter into the blender and blend until well combined.
- Heat 1 tablespoon of butter in a pan over medium heat.
- Pour some batter into a hot pan and swirl it around until evenly spread.
- Cook on medium heat until top has firmed up then flip and fry another side.
- Make crepes from remaining batter using the same method.
- Serve and enjoy.

Nutritional Value (Amount per Serving):

- Calories 139
- Fat 9.1 g
- Carbohydrates 11.8 g
- Sugar 0.4 g
- Protein 6.6 g
- Cholesterol 127 mg

Green Bean Summer Salad

Time: 20 minutes

Serve: 4

Ingredients:

- 1 lb green beans, trim and cut in half
- 2 cups cherry tomatoes, cut in half
- 1/2 onion, sliced
- 1/3 cup basil, sliced
- Pepper
- Salt
- For dressing:
- 1/2 tsp dried oregano
- 2 tsp garlic, minced
- 2 tbsp lemon juice
- 3 tbsp extra-virgin olive oil
- 1/2 tsp sea salt

Directions:

- Add beans in boiling water and cook for 5 minutes.
- Drain beans immediately and put them into the ice-cold water until cool.
- Drain beans from cold water and place in mixing bowl.
- Add cherry tomatoes, basil, and onion and toss well. Season with pepper and salt.
- In a small bowl, whisk together all dressing ingredients and pour over salad. Toss well.
- Serve and enjoy.

Nutritional Value (Amount per Serving):

- Calories 152
- Fat 10.9 g
- Carbohydrates 13 g
- Sugar 4.7 g
- Protein 3.2 g
- Cholesterol 0 mg

Parmesan Squash Noodles

Time: 30 minutes

Serve: 2

Ingredients:

- 1 medium butternut squash, peel and spiralized
- 1 tsp garlic powder
- 2 tbsp cream cheese
- 3 tbsp cream
- 1/4 cup parmesan cheese
- 1 tsp thyme, chopped
- 1 tbsp sage, chopped

Directions:

- Preheat the oven to 400 F/ 200 C.
- In a bowl, mix together cream cheese, parmesan, thyme, sage, cream, and garlic powder.
- Add noodles to a baking dish and bake for 20 minutes.
- Remove from oven and spread the cream cheese mixture over noodles and return to the oven and bake for 5 minutes.
- Serve and enjoy.

Nutritional Value (Amount per Serving):

- Calories 237
- Fat 15.8 g
- Carbohydrates 7.4 g
- Sugar 2.9 g
- Protein 17.6 g
- Cholesterol 43 mg

DAY 11

Delicious Zucchini Muffins

Time: 35 minutes

Serve: 8

Ingredients:

- 6 eggs
- 1/4 tsp ground nutmeg
- 1 tsp ground cinnamon
- 1/2 tsp baking soda
- 4 drops stevia
- 1/4 cup Swerve
- 1/3 cup coconut oil, melted
- 1 cup zucchini, grated
- 3/4 cup coconut flour

Directions:

- Preheat the oven to 356 F/ 180 C.
- Spray muffin tray with cooking spray and set aside.
- Add all ingredients except zucchini in a bowl and mix well.
- Add zucchini and stir well.
- Pour batter into the prepared muffin tray and bake in preheated oven for 25 minutes.
- Serve and enjoy.

Nutritional Value (Amount per Serving):

- Calories 135
- Fat 12.6 g
- Carbohydrates 1.8 g
- Sugar 0.6 g
- Protein 4.5 g
- Cholesterol 123 mg

Cucumber Cabbage Salad

Time: 20 minutes

Serve: 8

Ingredients:

- 2 cucumbers, sliced
- 3 tbsp olive oil
- 1/2 lemon juice
- 2 tbsp green onion, chopped
- 2 tbsp fresh dill, chopped
- 1/2 cabbage head, chopped
- Pepper
- Salt

Directions:

- Add cabbage to the mixing bowl. Season with 1 teaspoon of salt mix well and set aside.
- Add cucumbers, green onions, and fresh dill. Mix well.
- Add lemon juice, pepper, olive oil, and salt. Mix well.
- Place salad bowl in refrigerator for 1-2 hours.
- Serve chilled and enjoy.

Nutritional Value (Amount per Serving):

- Calories 71
- Fat 5.4 g
- Carbohydrates 5.9 g
- Sugar 2.8 g
- Protein 1.3 g
- Cholesterol 0 mg

Artichoke Cauliflower Couscous

Time: 25 minutes

Serve: 4

Ingredients:

- 1 head cauliflower, cut into florets
- 2 tbsp olive oil
- 1/4 cup parsley, chopped
- 1 lemon juice
- 14 black olives
- 1 garlic cloves, chopped
- 14 oz can artichokes
- 1/2 tsp pepper
- 1/2 tsp salt

Directions:

- Preheat the oven to 400 F/ 200 C.
- Add cauliflower florets into the food processor and process until it looks like rice.
- Spread cauliflower rice on a baking tray and drizzle with olive oil.
- Bake in preheated oven for 12 minutes.
- In a bowl, mix together garlic, lemon juice, artichokes, parsley, and olives.
- Add the cauliflower to the bowl and stir well.
- Season with pepper and salt.
- Serve and enjoy.

Nutritional Value (Amount per Serving):

- Calories 116
- Fat 8.8 g
- Carbohydrates 8.4 g
- Sugar 3.3 g
- Protein 3.3 g
- Cholesterol 0 mg

DAY 12

Perfect Mocha Smoothie

Time: 10 minutes

Serve: 3

Ingredients:

- 1 avocado, cut in half and pit removed
- 3 tbsp unsweetened cocoa powder
- 2 tsp instant coffee crystals
- 3 tbsp swerve
- 1 tsp vanilla extract
- 1 1/2 cups unsweetened almond milk
- 1/2 cup coconut milk

Directions:

- Add all ingredients to the blender and blend until smooth.
- Serve and enjoy.

Nutritional Value (Amount per Serving):

- Calories 199
- Fat 17.6 g
- Carbohydrates 12.4 g
- Sugar 0.6 g
- Protein 3.1 g
- Cholesterol 0 mg

Healthy Creamed Spinach

Time: 20 minutes

Serve: 4

Ingredients:

- 2 cups frozen spinach, thawed
- 1 tbsp lemon juice
- 1/2 cup coconut cream
- 1 tsp curry powder
- 2 garlic cloves, diced
- 1 large onion, sliced
- 1 tbsp coconut oil
- 2/3 tsp sea salt

Directions:

- Squeeze some excess liquid from spinach and roughly chop the spinach in half.
- Heat coconut oil in a pan over medium-high heat.
- Add onion and salt and sauté for 8 minutes or until softened.
- Add spinach, curry powder, and garlic and stir for a minute.
- Add lemon juice and coconut cream and stir until well combined.
- Serve and enjoy.

Nutritional Value (Amount per Serving):

- Calories 122
- Fat 10.8 g
- Carbohydrates 6.6 g
- Sugar 2.8 g
- Protein 1.7 g
- Cholesterol 0 mg

Feta Zucchini Frittata

Time: 30 minutes

Serve: 2

Ingredients:

- 5 eggs
- 2 tbsp olive oil
- 2 tbsp feta cheese, crumbled
- 2 tbsp fresh dill, chopped
- 2 tbsp sour cream
- 3 zucchinis, sliced
- 1/2 tsp pepper
- 1/2 tsp salt

Directions:

- Heat olive oil in a pan over medium heat.
- Add zucchini slices and cook for 10-15 minutes.
- Beat eggs in a bowl with sour cream and whisk until smooth.
- Add feta cheese, dill, and seasoning in egg mixture and mix well.
- Add egg mixture to the zucchini slices in the pan and cook for 8-10 minutes or until the bottom is firm.
- Serve and enjoy.

Nutritional Value (Amount per Serving):

- Calories 384
- Fat 30.1 g
- Carbohydrates 13.7 g
- Sugar 6.3 g
- Protein 19.8 g
- Cholesterol 423 mg

DAY 13

Moist Blueberry Muffins

Time: 30 minutes

Serve: 12

Ingredients:

- 3 large eggs
- 3/4 cup blueberries
- 1/2 tsp vanilla extract
- 1/3 cup unsweetened almond milk
- 1/3 cup coconut oil, melted
- 1 1/2 tsp gluten-free baking powder
- 1/2 cup erythritol
- 2 1/2 cups almond flour

Directions:

- Preheat the oven to 350 F/ 180 C.
- Spray muffin tray with cooking spray and set aside.
- In a large bowl, stir together almond flour, baking powder, erythritol.
- Mix in the coconut oil, vanilla, eggs, and almond milk. Fold in blueberries.
- Pour batter into the prepared muffin tray and bake in preheated oven for 20 minutes.
- Serve and enjoy.

Nutritional Value (Amount per Serving):

- Calories 217
- Fat 19 g
- Carbohydrates 6 g
- Protein 7 g
- Cholesterol 47 mg

Chili Garlic Mushrooms

Time: 25 minutes

Serve: 4

Ingredients:

- 2 tbsp lemon juice
- 3 garlic cloves, sliced
- 3 oz enoki mushrooms
- 1 tbsp butter
- 1 tsp lemon zest, chopped
- 6 oyster mushrooms, halved
- 5 oz cremini mushrooms, sliced
- 1/2 red chili, sliced
- 1/2 onion, sliced
- 2 tsp olive oil
- 1 tsp sea salt

Directions:

- Heat olive oil in a pan over high heat.
- Add shallots, enoki mushrooms, oyster mushrooms, cremini mushrooms, and chili. Stir well and cook over medium-high heat for 10 minutes.
- Add 1/2 tablespoon of butter halfway through.
- Add lemon zest and remaining butter and stir well. Season with lemon juice and salt and cook everything for 3-4 minutes.
- Serve and enjoy.

Nutritional Value (Amount per Serving):

- Calories 87
- Fat 5.6 g
- Carbohydrates 7.5 g
- Sugar 1.8 g
- Protein 3 g
- Cholesterol 8 mg

Feta Tomato Basil Frittata

Time: 25 minutes

Serve: 2

Ingredients:

- 5 eggs
- 1 tbsp olive oil
- 1/3 cup cherry tomatoes
- 2 tbsp fresh basil, chopped
- 1/4 cup feta cheese, crumbled
- 6.5 oz can artichokes
- 1 garlic clove, chopped
- 1 onion, chopped
- 1/4 tsp pepper
- 1/4 tsp salt

Directions:

- Heat oil in a pan over medium heat.
- Add garlic and onion and sauté for 4 minutes or until tender.
- Add artichokes, basil, and tomatoes and cook for 4 minutes.
- Beat eggs in a bowl and season with pepper and salt.
- Pour egg mixture into the pan and cook for 5-7 or until base firm.
- Serve and enjoy.

Nutritional Value (Amount per Serving):

- Calories 327
- Fat 22.1 g
- Carbohydrates 13.1 g
- Sugar 6.2 g
- Protein 19.1 g
- Cholesterol 426 mg

DAY 14

Quick and Healthy Smoothie Bowl

Time: 10 minutes

Serve: 1

Ingredients:

- 2 tbsp fresh lemon juice
- 1/4 cup ice cubes
- 1/4 cup erythritol
- 3/4 cup unsweetened coconut milk
- 1/2 medium avocado
- 1 cup spinach
- 1/2 scoop MCT oil powder
- 1/2 scoop perfect Keto collagen

Directions:

- Add all ingredients to the blender and blend until smooth.
- Pour green smoothie mixture into a bowl and top with coconut flakes and chia seeds.
- Serve and enjoy.

Nutritional Value (Amount per Serving):

- Calories 319
- Fat 26 g
- Carbohydrates 15 g
- Sugar 2 g
- Protein 10 g
- Cholesterol 0 mg

Lettuce Egg Cup

Time: 20 minutes

Serve: 6

Ingredients:

- 6 hard-boiled eggs, peel and slice in half
- 12 lettuce leaves
- 1/2 tsp garlic powder
- 2 tsp hot sauce
- 3 tbsp mayonnaise
- Pepper
- Salt

Directions:

- Arrange lettuce leaves on the platter and add egg halves on top of each lettuce leave.
- In a small bowl, combine together mayonnaise, garlic powder, and hot sauce and add a dollop on top of each egg.
- Season with pepper and salt.
- Serve and enjoy.

Nutritional Value (Amount per Serving):

- Calories 94
- Fat 6.9 g
- Carbohydrates 2.6 g
- Sugar 1 g
- Protein 5.7 g
- Cholesterol 166 mg

Broccoli Cheese Salad

Time: 10 minutes

Serve: 3

Ingredients:

- 4 cups broccoli florets
- 2 tbsp almond flakes
- 1/2 lemon juice
- 1 cup cherry tomatoes
- 2 tbsp mayonnaise
- 3.5 oz blue cheese, crumbled

Directions:

- In a small bowl, mash the blue cheese, mayonnaise, and lemon juice.
- Add broccoli florets and cherry tomatoes in a bowl.
- Add cheese mixture to broccoli and cherry tomatoes bowl and mix well.
- Add almond flakes and mix well.
- Cover salad bowl with lid and place in refrigerator for 30 minutes.
- Serve and enjoy.

Nutritional Value (Amount per Serving):

- Calories 123
- Fat 6.4 g
- Carbohydrates 13.3 g
- Sugar 4.3 g
- Protein 6.1 g
- Cholesterol 11 mg

DAY 15

Easy Pumpkin Muffins

Time: 35 minutes

Serve: 10

Ingredients:

- 4 large eggs
- 1 tsp vanilla extract
- 1/3 cup coconut oil, melted
- 1/2 cup pumpkin puree
- 1 tbsp pumpkin pie spice
- 1 tbsp gluten-free baking powder
- 2/3 cup erythritol
- 1/2 cup almond flour
- 1/2 cup coconut flour
- 1/2 tsp sea salt

Directions:

- Preheat the oven to 350 F/ 180 C.
- Spray muffin tray with cooking spray and set aside.
- In a large bowl, stir together coconut flour, pumpkin pie spice, baking powder, erythritol, almond flour, and sea salt.
- Stir in eggs, vanilla, coconut oil, and pumpkin puree until well combined.
- Pour batter into the prepared muffin tray and bake in preheated oven for 25 minutes.
- Serve and enjoy.

Nutritional Value (Amount per Serving):

- Calories 151
- Fat 13 g
- Carbohydrates 7 g
- Sugar 2 g
- Protein 5 g
- Cholesterol 74 mg

Cherry Tomato and Spinach Stir Fry

Time: 25 minutes

Serve: 2

Ingredients:

- 4 cups spinach
- 1 garlic clove, diced
- 1/2 tsp lemon zest
- 1/2 cup cherry tomatoes, cut in half
- 1/2 onion, sliced
- 2 tsp olive oil
- 6 button mushrooms, sliced
- 1 tsp butter
- Pepper
- Salt

Directions:

- Heat butter in a pan over medium heat.
- Add mushrooms and sauté for 3-4 minutes or until lightly browned.
- Remove mushrooms to a plate and set aside.
- Heat olive oil in the same pan over medium heat.
- Add onion and sauté for 2-3 minutes or until softened.
- Add tomatoes, garlic and lemon zest, and season with pepper and salt. Cook for 2-3 minutes and lightly smashed tomatoes with a spatula.
- Now add mushrooms and spinach and stir well and cook until spinach is wilted. Season with salt and drizzle with lemon juice.
- Serve and enjoy.

Nutritional Value (Amount per Serving):

- Calories 104
- Fat 7.1 g
- Carbohydrates 8.9 g
- Sugar 3.6 g
- Protein 4.3 g
- Cholesterol 5 mg

Parmesan Kale Frittata

Time: 25 minutes

Serve: 3

Ingredients:

- 4 eggs
- 2 tbsp olive oil
- 1 tbsp fresh sage, chopped
- 1/3 cup parmesan cheese, grated
- 4 cups kale, chopped
- 1/2 tsp pepper
- 1/2 tsp salt

Directions:

- Heat oil in a pan over medium heat.
- Add kale and cook for minutes or until wilted.
- In a bowl, beat eggs then add parmesan, sage, pepper, and salt.
- Pour egg mixture into the pan and cook for 8-10 minutes or until firm.
- Serve and enjoy.

Nutritional Value (Amount per Serving):

- Calories 411
- Fat 27.3 g
- Carbohydrates 10.4 g
- Sugar 0.5 g
- Protein 26.2 g
- Cholesterol 258 mg

DAY 16

Delicious Caprese Omelet

Time: 20 minutes

Serve: 2

Ingredients:

- 6 eggs
- 2 tbsp olive oil
- 5 oz mozzarella cheese, sliced
- 3 oz cherry tomatoes, cut in halves
- 1 tbsp fresh basil
- Pepper
- Salt

Directions:

- Add eggs in mixing bowl and season with pepper and salt. Whisk eggs with a fork until well combined.
- Stir in basil. Heat olive oil in a large pan over medium heat.
- Add tomatoes and sauté for few minutes.
- Pour eggs mixture on top of tomatoes and wait until eggs are slightly firm.
- Add mozzarella cheese slices on top and turn heat to low and let the omelet set.
- Serve and enjoy.

Nutritional Value (Amount per Serving):

- Calories 517
- Fat 39.7 g
- Carbohydrates 5.2 g
- Protein 37 g
- Cholesterol 529 mg

Radish Dill Salad

Time: 15 minutes

Serve: 4

Ingredients:

- 1 cucumber, sliced
- 3/4 cup light sour cream
- 2 tbsp chives, chopped
- 1/4 cup dill, chopped
- 10 radishes, sliced
- Pepper
- Salt

Directions:

- In a mixing bowl, combine the cucumber, dill, chives, and radishes.
- In a small bowl, combine together sour cream, pepper, and salt.
- Pour dressing over salad and toss everything well.
- Serve immediately and enjoy.

Nutritional Value (Amount per Serving):

- Calories 114
- Fat 9.3 g
- Carbohydrates 6.7 g
- Sugar 1.6 g
- Protein 2.6 g
- Cholesterol 19 mg

Delicious Tomato Soup

Time: 30 minutes

Serve: 4

Ingredients:

- 3 cups tomatoes, peeled, seeded and chopped
- 2 tbsp tomato paste
- 4 cups vegetable stock
- 1 tbsp garlic, minced
- 1 cup bell pepper, chopped
- 1 cup onion, chopped
- 1 tbsp olive oil
- 1/2 tsp thyme, chopped
- 1 tsp fresh oregano, chopped
- 1 tbsp basil, chopped
- 1/4 tsp pepper

Directions:

- Heat olive oil in large saucepan over medium heat.
- Add garlic, onion, bell pepper, and tomatoes and sauté for 10 minutes.
- Add all remaining ingredients and stir well to combine.
- Turn heat to high and bring to boil.
- Reduce heat to low and cover saucepan with lid and simmer for 10 minutes.
- Remove from heat and using blender puree the soup until smooth.
- Serve and enjoy.

Nutritional Value (Amount per Serving):

- Calories 97
- Fat 6 g
- Carbohydrates 14 g
- Sugar 9.3 g
- Protein 2.4 g
- Cholesterol 0 mg

DAY 17

Jalapeno Muffins

Time: 30 minutes

Serve: 8

Ingredients:

- 5 eggs
- 3 tbsp jalapenos, sliced
- 1/4 cup unsweetened coconut milk
- 1/3 cup coconut oil, melted
- 2 tsp baking powder
- 3 tbsp erythritol
- 2/3 cup coconut flour
- 3/4 tsp sea salt

Directions:

- Preheat the oven to 350 F/ 180 C.
- Spray muffin tray with cooking spray and set aside.
- In a large bowl, stir together coconut flour, baking powder, erythritol, and sea salt.
- Stir in eggs, jalapenos, coconut milk, and coconut oil until well combined.
- Pour batter into the prepared muffin tray and bake in preheated oven for 18-20 minutes.
- Serve and enjoy.

Nutritional Value (Amount per Serving):

- Calories 126
- Fat 12.1 g
- Carbohydrates 7.2 g
- Sugar 6 g
- Protein 3.7 g
- Cholesterol 102 mg

Salsa Stuffed Avocado

Time: 15 minutes

Serve: 4

Ingredients:

- 2 large avocado, cut in half and scooped
- 2 tbsp cilantro, chopped
- 1 lime juice
- 1 jalapeno pepper, diced
- 1/4 cup green onion, sliced
- 1 lb strawberries, diced
- Salt

Directions:

- In a bowl, mix together all ingredients except avocado.
- Stuff avocado with bowl mixture.
- Serve and enjoy.

Nutritional Value (Amount per Serving):

- Calories 142
- Fat 10.2 g
- Carbohydrates 13.7 g
- Sugar 6.1 g
- Protein 1.9 g
- Cholesterol 0 mg

Baked Zucchini Noodles

Time: 55 minutes

Serve: 3

Ingredients:

- 1 egg
- 2 medium zucchini, trimmed and spiralized
- 2 tbsp olive oil
- 1 cup mozzarella cheese, grated
- 1/2 cup parmesan cheese, grated
- 1/2 cup feta cheese, crumbled
- 1 tbsp thyme
- 1 garlic clove, chopped
- 1 onion, chopped
- 1/2 tsp pepper
- 1/2 tsp salt

Directions:

- Preheat the oven to 375 F/ 190 C.
- Add spiralized zucchini and salt in a colander and set aside for 10 minutes.
- Gently wash zucchini noodles and pat dry with paper towel.
- Heat oil in a pan over medium heat.
- Add garlic and onion and sauté for 3-4 minutes.
- Add zucchini noodles and cook for 4 minutes or until softened.
- Add zucchini mixture to a bowl add the eggs, thyme, cheeses. Mix well and season.
- Bake in preheated oven for 40-45 minutes.
- Serve and enjoy.

Nutritional Value (Amount per Serving):

- Calories 434
- Fat 30.2 g
- Carbohydrates 10.4 g
- Sugar 5 g
- Protein 26.3 g
- Cholesterol 122 mg

DAY 18

Easy Egg Scrambled

Time: 15 minutes

Serve: 4

Ingredients:

- 6 eggs
- 2 tbsp butter
- 3 oz shredded cheese
- 1 tomato, chopped
- 2 pickled jalapenos, chopped
- 1 scallion, chopped
- Pepper
- Salt

Directions:

- Melt butter in a pan over medium heat.
- Add tomatoes, jalapenos, and scallions and sauté for 3 minutes.
- Beat eggs in a bowl and pour into the pan and scramble for 2 minutes.
- Add cheese and stir well. Season with pepper and salt.
- Serve and enjoy.

Nutritional Value (Amount per Serving):

- Calories 235
- Fat 19.4 g
- Carbohydrates 1.7 g
- Sugar 1.1 g
- Protein 13.9 g
- Cholesterol 283 mg

Garlic Roasted Carrots

Time: 45 minutes

Serve: 6

Ingredients:

- 6 garlic cloves, minced
- 16 small carrots
- 1 tbsp fresh parsley, chopped
- 1 tbsp dried basil
- 4 tbsp olive oil
- 1 1/2 tsp salt

Directions:

- Preheat the oven to 190 C/ 375 F.
- In a bowl, combine together oil, carrots, basil, garlic, and salt.
- Spread the carrots onto a baking tray and bake in preheated oven for 35 minutes.
- Garnish with parsley and serve.

Nutritional Value (Amount per Serving):

- Calories 139
- Fat 9.4 g
- Carbohydrates 14.2 g
- Sugar 6.6 g
- Protein 1.3 g
- Cholesterol 0 mg

Spinach Cauliflower Risotto

Time: 30 minutes

Serve: 2

Ingredients:

- 1 cauliflower head, cut into florets
- 1 tbsp olive oil
- 1/2 cup vegetable stock
- 1/2 cup parmesan cheese, grated
- 2 tbsp heavy cream
- 1 small onion, chopped
- 1 cup fresh spinach, chopped
- 1/2 tsp black pepper
- 1/2 tsp salt

Directions:

- Add cauliflower florets into the food processor and process until it looks like rice.
- Heat oil in a pan over medium heat.
- Add onion and sauté for 5 minutes or until tender.
- Add cauliflower rice and toss to coat in the oil.
- Add spinach and stock; simmer on low heat for about 10 minutes or until tender.
- Add cheese and cream and stir well and season. Cook for 2-3 minutes more or until cheese has melted.
- Serve and enjoy.

Nutritional Value (Amount per Serving):

- Calories 466
- Fat 31.3 g
- Carbohydrates 12.1 g
- Sugar 5.2 g
- Protein 27.8 g
- Cholesterol 81 mg

DAY 19

Blueberry Breakfast Smoothie

Time: 10 minutes

Serve: 2

Ingredients:

- 1/2 cup fresh blueberries
- 1/2 tsp vanilla extract
- 1 tbsp lemon juice
- 14 oz coconut milk

Directions:

- Add all ingredients to the blender and blend until smooth.
- Serve and enjoy.

Nutritional Value (Amount per Serving):

- Calories 58
- Fat 3.6 g
- Carbohydrates 6.3 g
- Sugar 4.4 g
- Protein 0.7 g
- Cholesterol 0 mg

Creamy Mushrooms

Time: 45 minutes

Serve: 4

Ingredients:

- 1 1/2 lbs mushrooms, cleaned and quartered
- 1/2 cup heavy whipping cream
- 1/2 cup dry red wine
- 1 tbsp dried basil
- 2 garlic cloves, minced
- 1 onion, sliced
- 2 tbsp butter
- 1/2 tsp black pepper
- 1 1/2 tsp salt

Directions:

- Heat butter in a large pan over medium-high heat.
- Add onion and sauté for 15 minutes or until softened.
- Add mushrooms and season with pepper and salt and cook for another 15 minutes.
- Add basil and garlic and stir well.
- Add wine and stir well. Turn heat to low and continue to reduce wine over low heat.
- Add cream and stir for a minute.
- Serve and enjoy.

Nutritional Value (Amount per Serving):

- Calories 178
- Fat 11.9 g
- Carbohydrates 10.1 g
- Sugar 4.4 g
- Protein 6.2 g
- Cholesterol 36 mg

Basil Zucchini Soup

Time: 25 minutes

Serve: 4

Ingredients:

- 2 large zucchini, trimmed and cut into chunks
- 1/3 cup basil leaves
- 3 cups vegetable stock
- 2 tbsp coconut oil
- 2 garlic cloves, chopped
- 1 onion, chopped
- Pepper
- Salt

Directions:

- Heat coconut oil in a large saucepan over medium heat.
- Add garlic and onion and sauté for 3-5 minutes or until softened.
- Add zucchini and cook for 5 minutes. Stir occasionally.
- Add vegetable stock, bring to boil and simmer for 15 minutes.
- Add basil and puree the soup using a blender until smooth.
- Season with pepper and salt.
- Serve and enjoy.

Nutritional Value (Amount per Serving):

- Calories 101
- Fat 7.6 g
- Carbohydrates 9.1 g
- Sugar 4.5 g
- Protein 2.4 g
- Cholesterol 0 mg

DAY 20

Coconut Ginger Smoothie

Time: 10 minutes

Serve: 2

Ingredients:

- 2 tsp fresh ginger, grated
- 1 oz spinach
- 2 tbsp lime juice
- 2/3 cup water
- 1/3 cup coconut milk

Directions:

- Add all ingredients to the blender and blend until smooth.
- Serve immediately and enjoy.

Nutritional Value (Amount per Serving):

- Calories 105
- Fat 9.8 g
- Carbohydrates 5 g
- Sugar 1.7 g
- Protein 1.5 g
- Cholesterol 0 mg

Garlic Carrot Salad

Time: 40 minutes

Serve: 4

Ingredients:

- 8 medium carrots, peeled and julienne
- 2 tbsp fresh cilantro
- 1/4 tsp cumin
- 2 tbsp apple cider vinegar
- 5 garlic cloves
- 1 onion
- 3 tbsp avocado oil
- 2 tsp sea salt

Directions:

- Add carrots julienne and salt in a mixing bowl. Toss well and set aside.
- Heat oil in a pan over medium heat.
- Add onion and cook until lightly golden brown.
- While onion is cooking, add garlic, cumin, and apple cider vinegar to the carrots. Mix well and set aside.
- Once onion is done, allow to cool. Once onion is cooked, combine with carrots and toss well.
- Garnish with cilantro and serve.

Nutritional Value (Amount per Serving):

- Calories 159
- Fat 10.6 g
- Carbohydrates 14 g
- Sugar 7.2 g
- Protein 1.6 g
- Cholesterol 0 mg

Spicy Cabbage Soup

Time: 35 minutes

Serve: 4

Ingredients:

- 1 small cabbage head
- 2 tbsp coconut oil
- 3 cups vegetable stock
- 1/4 cup coconut milk
- 1 tsp cumin powder
- 2 tsp turmeric powder
- 2 garlic cloves, chopped
- 1/2 tsp black pepper
- 1/2 tsp salt

Directions:

- Heat coconut oil in a saucepan over medium heat.
- Add cabbage and garlic and sauté for 10 minutes or until cabbage is softened.
- Add stock and stir well. Bring to boil and simmer for 20 minutes.
- Remove from heat and add coconut milk and spices. Stir well.
- Using blender puree the soup until smooth and creamy.
- Serve and enjoy.

Nutritional Value (Amount per Serving):

- Calories 149
- Fat 11.3 g
- Carbohydrates 13.3 g
- Sugar 6.8 g
- Protein 2.9 g
- Cholesterol 0 mg

DAY 21

Mushroom Spinach Frittata

Time: 15 minutes

Serve: 1

Ingredients:

- 1 cup egg whites
- 2 tbsp parmesan cheese, grated
- 1 cup spinach, chopped
- 2 mushrooms, sliced
- Salt

Directions:

- Spray 7-inch pan with cooking spray and heat over medium heat.
- Add mushrooms and sauté for 2-3 minutes.
- Add spinach and cook for 1-2 minutes or until wilted.
- Whisk egg whites in a mixing bowl until frothy. Season with a pinch of salt.
- Pour egg white mixture into the spinach and mushroom mixture and sprinkle with parmesan cheese. Let cook for 1-2 minutes.
- Transfer frittata to the frying pan and broil in preheated oven for 2-3 minutes.
- Cut into wedges and serve.

Nutritional Value (Amount per Serving):

- Calories 178
- Fat 2.9 g
- Carbohydrates 4 g
- Sugar 2.5 g
- Protein 31.5 g
- Cholesterol 8 mg

Dill Turnip Salad

Time: 10 minutes

Serve: 4

Ingredients:

- 4 white turnips, spiralized
- 2 tbsp olive oil
- 1 lemon juice
- 4 dill sprigs, chopped
- 1 1/2 tsp salt

Directions:

- Season spiralized turnip with salt and gently massage with hands.
- Add lemon juice and dill. Season with pepper and salt.
- Drizzle with olive oil and combine everything well.
- Serve immediately and enjoy.

Nutritional Value (Amount per Serving):

- Calories 49
- Fat 1.1 g
- Carbohydrates 9 g
- Sugar 5.2 g
- Protein 1.4 g
- Cholesterol 0 mg

Creamy Zucchini Fennel Soup

Time: 25 minutes

Serve: 4

Ingredients:

- 2 zucchinis, chopped
- 2 fennel bulbs, chopped
- 1 tsp coconut oil
- 2 cups vegetable stock
- 1/4 tsp fennel seeds
- 1 onion, chopped
- Pepper
- Salt

Directions:

- Heat oil in a large saucepan over medium heat.
- Add fennel seed and onion and sauté for 3 minutes.
- Add zucchini and fennel and cook for 5 minutes.
- Add stock and stir well. Bring to boil then cover and simmer for 15 minutes.
- Using blender puree the soup until smooth and creamy. Season with pepper and salt.
- Serve and enjoy.

Nutritional Value (Amount per Serving):

- Calories 78
- Fat 2.6 g
- Carbohydrates 14 g
- Sugar 3.9 g
- Protein 3 g
- Cholesterol 0 mg

DAY 22

Avocado Strawberry Smoothie

Time: 10 minutes

Serve: 5

Ingredients:

- 1 avocado
- 1 1/2 cups unsweetened almond milk
- 1 lb strawberries
- 1/4 cup erythritol

Directions:

- Add all ingredients to the blender and blend until smooth.
- Serve and enjoy.

Nutritional Value (Amount per Serving):

- Calories 106
- Fat 7 g
- Carbohydrates 12 g
- Sugar 4 g
- Protein 1 g
- Cholesterol 0 mg

Refreshing Cucumber Salad

Time: 20 minutes

Serve: 6

Ingredients:

- 6 cucumbers, sliced
- 1 tsp sesame seeds
- 1/2 tsp red pepper flakes
- 2 tbsp fresh cilantro, chopped
- 1 tbsp coconut aminos
- 2 tbsp sesame oil
- 2 tbsp vinegar
- 1/4 onion, sliced
- 1 tsp salt

Directions:

- Add cucumbers and onion to the mixing bowl and mix well.
- In a small bowl, combine together remaining ingredients and mix well.
- Pour dressing over cucumber and onion and combine everything well.
- Serve immediately and enjoy.

Nutritional Value (Amount per Serving):

- Calories 92
- Fat 5.1 g
- Carbohydrates 11.6 g
- Sugar 5.3 g
- Protein 2.1 g
- Cholesterol 0 mg

Cheese Jalapeno Cauliflower Soup

Time: 30 minutes

Serve: 4

Ingredients:

- 1 cauliflower head, cut into florets
- 2 tbsp olive oil
- 2 cups cheddar cheese, grated
- 1/2 tsp garlic powder
- 2 cups vegetable stock
- 4 jalapeno peppers, chopped
- 3 garlic cloves, chopped
- 1 onion, chopped
- Pepper
- Salt

Directions:

- Heat olive oil in a large saucepan over medium heat.
- Add onions, garlic, and jalapeno and sauté for 5 minutes or until softened.
- Add cauliflower and sauté for 2 minutes.
- Add garlic powder and stock, bring to boil then simmer for 20 minutes or until cauliflower is tender.
- Add cheddar cheese and season with pepper and salt. Cook for 5 minutes more until cheese has melted.
- Serve and enjoy.

Nutritional Value (Amount per Serving):

- Calories 328
- Fat 26.5 g
- Carbohydrates 9.4 g
- Sugar 4.1 g
- Protein 16.1 g
- Cholesterol 59 mg

DAY 23

Spinach Egg Breakfast Casserole

Time: 45 minutes

Serve: 6

Ingredients:

- 2 eggs
- 1 1/4 cup cheddar cheese, shredded
- 1/2 red pepper, chopped
- 1/2 green pepper, chopped
- 1/2 onion, chopped
- 1 cup mushrooms, sliced
- 2 cups frozen spinach, thawed and drained
- 1 1/2 cups egg whites
- Pepper
- Salt

Directions:

- Preheat the oven to 375 F/ 176 C.
- Spray casserole dish with cooking spray.
- Heat pan over medium-high heat.
- Add chopped vegetables except spinach to the pan and sauté for few minutes until vegetables are soft.
- Add vegetables to the bottom of casserole dish and spread the vegetables to the dish.
- Add spinach to the vegetables and spread well.
- Whisk eggs and egg whites in a small bowl and season with pepper and salt.
- Pour egg mixture over the vegetables. Sprinkle with shredded cheese.
- Bake in preheated oven for 35 minutes.
- Serve and enjoy.

Nutritional Value (Amount per Serving):

- Calories 161
- Fat 9.5 g
- Carbohydrates 3.7 g
- Sugar 2 g
- Protein 15.3 g
- Cholesterol 79 mg

Cabbage Avocado Salad

Time: 20 minutes

Serve: 4

Ingredients:

- 2 avocados, diced
- 4 cups cabbage, shredded
- 3 tbsp fresh parsley, chopped
- 2 tbsp apple cider vinegar
- 4 tbsp avocado oil
- 1 cup cherry tomatoes, halved
- 1/2 tsp pepper
- 1 1/2 tsp sea salt

Directions:

- Add cabbage, avocados, and tomatoes to a medium bowl and mix well.
- In a small bowl, whisk together oil, parsley, vinegar, pepper, and salt.
- Pour dressing over vegetables and mix well.
- Serve immediately and enjoy.

Nutritional Value (Amount per Serving):

- Calories 253
- Fat 21.6 g
- Carbohydrates 14 g
- Sugar 4 g
- Protein 3.5 g
- Cholesterol 0 mg

Cauliflower Broccoli Soup

Time: 25 minutes

Serve: 2

Ingredients:

- 2 cups broccoli, cut into florets
- 1/2 cauliflower head, cut into florets
- 1 tbsp olive oil
- 2 cups vegetable stock
- 1 garlic clove, chopped
- 1 small onion, chopped
- Pepper
- Salt

Directions:

- Preheat the oven to 350 F/ 180 C.
- Place cauliflower and broccoli on a baking tray and drizzle with olive oil. Roast in preheated oven for 30 minutes.
- Sauté garlic and onion in a saucepan for 5-6 minutes or until softened.
- Add broccoli, cauliflower, and stock. Bring to boil and simmer for 15 minutes.
- Puree the soup using an immersion blender until smooth and creamy.
- Serve and enjoy.

Nutritional Value (Amount per Serving):

- Calories 129
- Fat 8.4 g
- Carbohydrates 14.4 g
- Sugar 5.6 g
- Protein 4.4 g
- Cholesterol 0 mg

DAY 24

Ginger Avocado Smoothie

Time: 10 minutes

Serve: 2

Ingredients:

- 1/2 avocado
- 1 cup ice cube, crushed
- 1 tsp fresh lemon juice
- 1/2 tsp turmeric
- 1 tsp ginger, grated
- 1/4 cup almond milk
- 3/4 cup coconut milk

Directions:

- Add all ingredients to the blender and blend until smooth.
- Serve immediately and enjoy.

Nutritional Value (Amount per Serving):

- Calories 224
- Fat 21.6 g
- Carbohydrates 8.1 g
- Sugar 1.4 g
- Protein 2.3 g
- Cholesterol 0 mg

Healthy Coconut Cabbage Salad

Time: 10 minutes

Serve: 3

Ingredients:

- 1/2 head cabbage, shredded
- 1/2 tsp cumin
- 1/2 tsp curry powder
- 1/2 tsp ginger, dried
- 3 tsp sesame seeds
- 1/4 cup tamari sauce
- 1/4 cup coconut oil
- 1 lemon juice
- 1/3 cup unsweetened desiccated coconut

Directions:

- Add all ingredients into the mixing bowl and mix well.
- Place salad bowl in refrigerator for 1 hour.
- Serve chilled and enjoy.

Nutritional Value (Amount per Serving):

- Calories 296
- Fat 29 g
- Carbohydrates 9.8 g
- Sugar 4.6 g
- Protein 4.8 g
- Cholesterol 0 mg

Easy Spinach Pie

Time: 35 minutes

Serve: 6

Ingredients:

- 5 eggs, beaten
- 2 1/2 cups cheese, grated
- 10 oz frozen spinach, thawed, squeezed, and drained
- 1/4 tsp garlic powder
- 1 tsp dried onion, minced
- Pepper
- Salt

Directions:

- Spray a 9-inch pie dish with cooking spray and set aside.
- Add all ingredients into the mixing bowl and mix until well combined.
- Pour pie mixture into the prepared dish and bake at 375 F/ 190 C for 30 minutes.
- Serve and enjoy.

Nutritional Value (Amount per Serving):

- Calories 254
- Fat 19.4 g
- Carbohydrates 2.8 g
- Sugar 0.8 g
- Protein 17.7 g
- Cholesterol 186 mg

DAY 25

Warm Coconut Porridge

Time: 10 minutes

Serve: 1

Ingredients:

- 1 egg, beaten
- 1 tbsp swerve
- 1 tbsp heavy cream
- 2 tsp butter
- 3/4 cup water
- 2 tbsp golden flax meal
- 2 tbsp coconut flour
- Pinch of salt

Directions:

- Add coconut flour, salt, water, and golden flax meal into a small pot and heat over medium heat. Stir well.
- Once it begins to simmer then turn heat medium-low and whisk until thickened.
- Remove pot from heat and add beaten egg and whisk continuously.
- Return pot on a heat and whisk until porridge thickens.
- Remove from heat and continue whisk for 30 seconds before adding sweetener, cream, and butter.
- Garnish with your favorite toppings and serve.

Nutritional Value (Amount per Serving):

- Calories 453
- Fat 39 g
- Carbohydrates 14 g
- Sugar 0.4 g
- Protein 10.9 g
- Cholesterol 204 mg

Spinach Zucchini Noodles

Time: 25 minutes

Serves: 4

Ingredients:

- 2 medium zucchini, spiralized into noodles
- 1 tbsp olive oil
- 1/3 cup parmesan cheese, grated
- 4 oz cream cheese
- 1 cup spinach
- 1/2 cup basil leaves
- 2 garlic cloves, chopped
- 1/2 tsp black pepper
- 1/2 tsp salt

Directions:

- Heat oil in a saucepan over medium heat.
- Add garlic and sauté for 3-5 minutes or until lightly golden brown.
- Add zucchini noodles and cook for 8-10 minutes.
- Stir in cream cheese, basil, and spinach and stir until cream cheese has become a sauce.
- Add parmesan cheese and season with pepper and salt.
- Serve and enjoy.

Nutritional Value (Amount per Serving):

- Calories 174
- Fat 15.2 g
- Carbohydrates 5.1 g
- Sugar 1.8 g
- Protein 6.4 g
- Cholesterol 37 mg

Yummy Spinach Mushrooms Pie

Time: 55 minutes

Serve: 4

Ingredients:

- 4 eggs
- 1 1/2 cups cheddar cheese, grated
- 3 oz cream cheese, softened
- 8 oz spinach leaves
- 1/4 cup butter
- 12 mushrooms, sliced
- 1 tsp garlic, minced
- 1/2 onion, chopped

Directions:

- Heat butter in a pan over medium heat.
- Add onion, mushrooms, and garlic and sauté until softened.
- Add spinach and cook until spinach is wilted.
- In a medium bowl, whisk eggs until frothy. Add cream cheese and whisk again for a minute.
- Add veggies and one cup grated cheese.
- Pour the mixture into a greased casserole dish and cover with remaining cheese.
- Bake at 350 F for 45 minutes or until lightly browned.
- Serve and enjoy.

Nutritional Value (Amount per Serving):

- Calories 441
- Fat 37.7 g
- Carbohydrates 6.8 g
- Sugar 2.4 g
- Protein 21.3 g
- Cholesterol 262 mg

DAY 26

Delicious Turmeric Scrambled Egg

Time: 10 minutes

Serve: 2

Ingredients:

- 4 large eggs
- 1/2 tsp dried parsley
- 2 tsp turmeric
- 2 tbsp coconut milk
- Pepper
- Salt

Directions:

- Spray a small pan with cooking spray and heat over medium heat.
- In a small bowl, whisk together eggs, parsley, turmeric, milk, pepper, and salt.
- Transfer eggs mixture to the hot pan and cook for 2-3 minutes. Stir eggs constantly.
- Stir well and cook for 2-3 minutes more.
- Serve and enjoy.

Nutritional Value (Amount per Serving):

- Calories 186
- Fat 13.7 g
- Carbohydrates 3.1 g
- Sugar 1.3 g
- Protein 13.1 g
- Cholesterol 372 mg

Arugula Halloumi Salad

Time: 15 minutes

Serves: 3

Ingredients:

- 1 tbsp olive oil
- 2 cups arugula
- 6 strawberries, sliced
- 7.5 oz halloumi cheese, cubed
- 1 avocado, chopped
- For dressing:
- 1 tbsp mint, chopped
- 1 tbsp basil, chopped
- 2 tbsp olive oil
- 1 tbsp lime juice
- 1/2 tsp pepper
- 1/2 tsp salt

Directions:

- Heat 1 tablespoon of oil in a pan over medium heat.
- Add cheese to the oil and cook until all sides are lightly golden. Set aside.
- In a small bowl, whisk together all dressing ingredients.
- In a large bowl place the arugula and then scatter the cheese, avocado, and strawberries.
- Pour dressing over the salad and toss to coat.
- Serve immediately and enjoy.

Nutritional Value (Amount per Serving):

- Calories 528
- Fat 48.4 g
- Carbohydrates 10.3 g
- Sugar 3.6 g
- Protein 17.2 g
- Cholesterol 56 mg

Parmesan Eggplant Bites

Time: 25 minutes

Serve: 5

Ingredients:

- 1 eggplant, sliced
- 1 egg
- Pepper
- Salt
- 1/4 cup parmesan cheese, grated
- 1/2 cup cheese, grated
- 1/2 tbsp dried rosemary
- 1/2 tbsp dried thyme
- 1/4 cup almond flour

Directions:

- Place sliced eggplants on a baking tray and season with pepper and salt. Bake at 350 F/ 180 C until lightly browned.
- In a small bowl, mix together almond flour, dried rosemary, dried thyme, and grated cheese.
- Remove eggplant slice from oven and season with pepper and salt.
- Return to the oven and cook until lightly browned.
- Remove from oven and brush with beaten egg.
- Sprinkle with almond flour mixture and bake until cheese is melted.
- Serve and enjoy.

Nutritional Value (Amount per Serving):

- Calories 145
- Fat 9.4 g
- Carbohydrates 7.2 g
- Sugar 3.1 g
- Protein 8.5 g
- Cholesterol 51 mg

DAY 27

Creamy Cauliflower Mashed

Time: 4 hours 5 minutes

Serve: 6

Ingredients:

- 1 medium cauliflower head, cut into florets
- 1/4 tsp onion powder
- 1/2 tsp dried parsley
- 1 tsp dried dill weed
- 2 garlic cloves, minced
- 1/4 cup butter
- 1/3 cup sour cream
- 1/2 tsp pepper
- 3/4 tsp sea salt

Directions:

- Add all ingredients to a slow cooker and stir well.
- Seal slow cooker with lid and cook on low for 4 hours.
- Transfer cauliflower mixture to a blender and blend until smooth.
- Serve and enjoy.

Nutritional Value (Amount per Serving):

- Calories 122
- Fat 10.5 g
- Carbohydrates 6.3 g
- Sugar 2.4 g
- Protein 2.5 g
- Cholesterol 26 mg

Mix Veggies Salad

Time: 15 minutes

Serves: 6

Ingredients:

- 1 bell pepper, seeded and chopped
- 1 cucumber, seeded and chopped
- 2 cups cauliflower florets
- 2 cups carrots, chopped
- 2 cups cherry tomatoes, halved
- 2 tbsp shallots, minced
- For dressing:
- 2 garlic cloves, minced
- 1/2 cup red wine vinegar
- 1/2 cup olive oil
- Pepper
- Salt

Directions:

- In a small bowl, combine together all dressing ingredients.
- Add all salad ingredients to the large bowl and toss well.
- Pour dressing over salad and toss well.
- Place salad bowl in refrigerator for 3-4 hours.
- Serve chilled and enjoy.

Nutritional Value (Amount per Serving):

- Calories 200
- Fat 17.1 g
- Carbohydrates 12.1 g
- Protein 2.2 g
- Cholesterol 0 mg

Mushroom Spinach Cheese Quiche

Time: 45 minutes

Serve: 6

Ingredients:

- 6 eggs
- 1 cup mozzarella cheese, shredded
- 1/2 tsp garlic powder
- 1/3 cup parmesan cheese, shredded
- 1/2 cup water
- 1/2 cup heavy cream
- 2 cheese slices
- 8 oz can mushroom, sliced
- 10 oz frozen spinach, thawed and drained
- Pepper
- Salt

Directions:

- Spread spinach into a pie pan and spread mushrooms over spinach.
- Whisk eggs together with water and heavy cream. Mix in garlic powder, parmesan, pepper, and salt.
- Pour egg mixture over other ingredients in pie pan. Top with shredded mozzarella cheese.
- Bake at 350 F for 40 minutes or until lightly golden brown.
- Serve and enjoy.

Nutritional Value (Amount per Serving):

- Calories 186
- Fat 13.4 g
- Carbohydrates 4.2 g
- Sugar 0.7 g
- Protein 13.1 g
- Cholesterol 193 mg

DAY 28

Jalapeno Cheddar Biscuits

Time: 30 minutes

Serve: 8

Ingredients:

- 1 large egg
- 1/4 cup pickled jalapeno, chopped
- 1/4 cup water
- 1/4 cup heavy cream
- 1 1/4 cups almond flour
- 1/4 tsp onion powder
- 1/4 tsp garlic powder
- 1/4 tsp Italian seasoning
- 3 garlic cloves, minced
- 1 1/2 cups cheddar cheese, shredded
- 4 oz cream cheese, softened

Directions:

- Preheat the oven to 350 F/ 180 C.
- Spray muffin pan with cooking spray and set aside.
- Beat egg and cream cheese in a bowl until well combined.
- Add cheddar cheese, onion powder, garlic powder, Italian seasoning, and garlic and mix well.
- Mix in almond flour, jalapeno, water, and heavy cream.
- Pour batter into the prepared muffin pan and bake in preheated oven for 20 minutes.
- Serve and enjoy.

Nutritional Value (Amount per Serving):

- Calories 260
- Fat 22.8 g
- Carbohydrates 5.2 g
- Sugar 1 g
- Protein 11.1 g
- Cholesterol 66 mg

Easy Avocado Egg Salad

Time: 10 minutes

Serve: 4

Ingredients:

- 1 avocado, mashed
- 8 hard-boiled eggs, chopped
- 1/2 tsp sea salt
- 2 tbsp fresh lemon juice

Directions:

- In a large bowl combine together avocado, eggs, sea salt and lemon juice.
- Toss well until combined.
- Serve immediately and enjoy.

Nutritional Value (Amount per Serving):

- Calories 230
- Fat 18.6 g
- Carbohydrates 5.2 g
- Sugar 1.1 g
- Protein 12.1 g
- Cholesterol 327 mg

Creamy Onion Soup

Time: 45 minutes

Serve: 4

Ingredients:

- 1 onion, sliced
- 4 cups vegetable broth
- 1 garlic clove, chopped
- 1 leek, sliced
- 1 1/2 tbsp olive oil
- 1 shallot, sliced
- Salt

Directions:

- Add broth and olive oil in a saucepan and bring to boil.
- Add remaining ingredients and stir well.
- Cover pan and simmer for 25 minutes.
- Using blender puree the soup until smooth and creamy.
- Serve and enjoy.

Nutritional Value (Amount per Serving):

- Calories 109
- Fat 6.7 g
- Carbohydrates 6.9 g
- Sugar 2.8 g
- Protein 5.5 g
- Cholesterol 0 mg

DAY 29

Easy Cappuccino Muffins

Time: 45 minutes

Serve: 12

Ingredients:

- 4 eggs
- 1 tsp cinnamon
- 2 tsp baking powder
- 1/4 cup coconut flour
- 1/2 cup Swerve
- 2 cups almond flour
- 1/2 tsp vanilla
- 1 tsp espresso powder
- 1/2 cup sour cream
- 1/4 tsp salt

Directions:

- Preheat the oven to 350 F/ 176 C.
- Spray muffin tray with cooking spray and set aside.
- Add sour cream, vanilla, espresso powder, and eggs in a blender and blend until smooth.
- Add almond flour, cinnamon, baking powder, coconut flour, sweetener, and salt. Blend again until smooth.
- Pour mixture into the prepared muffin tray and bake in preheated oven for 23-25 minutes.
- Serve and enjoy.

Nutritional Value (Amount per Serving):

- Calories 151
- Fat 12.9 g
- Carbohydrates 5.3 g
- Sugar 0.8 g
- Protein 6.2 g
- Cholesterol 59 mg

Asparagus with Mushrooms

Time: 10 minutes

Serve: 4

Ingredients:

- 1 lb asparagus, trimmed and cut into pieces
- 1/4 cup water
- 12 mushrooms, sliced
- 3 tbsp butter
- Pepper
- Salt

Directions:

- In a large pan, melt the butter over medium heat.
- Add mushroom and salt and sauté for 1 minute or until mushroom is golden brown.
- Remove mushrooms to plate and add asparagus season with pepper and salt.
- Cook asparagus for 2 minutes or until softened.
- Remove from heat and mix with mushrooms.
- Serve and enjoy.

Nutritional Value (Amount per Serving):

- Calories 111
- Fat 8.9 g
- Carbohydrates 6.2 g
- Sugar 3.1 g
- Protein 4.3 g
- Cholesterol 23 mg

Mushroom Cauliflower Risotto

Time: 40 minutes

Serve: 6

Ingredients:

- 4 cups cauliflower florets
- 2 tbsp parsley, chopped
- 1/2 cup parmesan cheese, grated
- 1 cup heavy cream
- 2 cups vegetable stock
- 8 oz cremini mushrooms, sliced
- 1 large shallot, minced
- 1 small onion, diced
- 6 garlic cloves, minced
- 2 tbsp olive oil
- 2 tbsp butter
- Pepper
- Salt

Directions:

- Heat oil and butter in a pan over medium heat.
- Add shallot, onion, and garlic and sauté until softened, about 5 minutes.
- Add mushrooms and 1 cup vegetable stock. Sauté until mushrooms soften, about 5 minutes.
- Add cauliflower and remaining stock and stir frequently and cook for 10 minutes.
- Turn heat to low and stir in parmesan cheese, heavy cream, parsley, pepper, and salt. Simmer for 10-15 minutes to thicken.
- Serve and enjoy.

Nutritional Value (Amount per Serving):

- Calories 283
- Fat 22.7 g
- Carbohydrates 8.5 g
- Sugar 3.5 g
- Protein 11.1 g
- Cholesterol 58 mg

DAY 30

Healthy Chia Blueberry Smoothie

Time: 10 minutes

Serve: 4

Ingredients:

- 1 cup blueberries
- 2 tbsp swerve
- 2 tbsp chia seed
- 2 tbsp coconut oil
- 1 cup unsweetened almond milk
- 1/2 cup coconut cream
- 1 cup coconut milk

Directions:

- Add all ingredients to the blender and blend until smooth.
- Serve and enjoy.

Nutritional Value (Amount per Serving):

- Calories 249
- Fat 21 g
- Carbohydrates 11 g
- Sugar 4.6 g
- Protein 6.2 g
- Cholesterol 18 mg

Cheesy Egg with Pepper

Time: 10 minutes

Serve: 4

Ingredients:

- 4 eggs
- 1/4 cup parmesan cheese, grated
- 1 bell pepper
- 1 tbsp olive oil
- Pepper
- Salt

Directions:

- Heat olive oil in a pan over medium heat.
- Cut bell pepper into 1/2 inch rings and place in the pan.
- Sauté peppers for 1 minute. Add 1 egg into the center of each pepper slice. Pour gently.
- Season with pepper and salt and cook for 3 minutes, then turn it carefully.
- Sprinkle with grated parmesan cheese and cook for a minute.
- Serve and enjoy.

Nutritional Value (Amount per Serving):

- Calories 140
- Fat 10.2 g
- Carbohydrates 2.6 g
- Sugar 1.8 g
- Protein 8.8 g
- Cholesterol 171 mg

Broccoli Casserole

Time: 40 minutes

Serve: 8

Ingredients:

- 2 lbs broccoli florets
- 2 garlic cloves, minced
- 4 oz cream cheese
- 1 cup mozzarella cheese
- 2 cups cheddar cheese, shredded
- 1/4 cup vegetable stock
- 1/2 cup heavy cream
- 3 tbsp olive oil
- Pepper
- Salt

Directions:

- Preheat the oven to 400 F/ 204 C.
- Layer broccoli florets in a casserole dish. Drizzle with olive oil and season with pepper and salt.
- Roast broccoli in preheated oven for 15-20 minutes.
- Meanwhile, combine together heavy cream, stock, garlic, cream cheese, mozzarella cheese, and 1 cup cheddar cheese in a medium saucepan over medium-low heat. Stir frequently.
- Once broccoli is cooked then pour heavy cream mixture over top and mix everything well.
- Sprinkle remaining cheddar cheese on top and bake in preheated oven for 15 minutes more.
- Serve and enjoy.

Nutritional Value (Amount per Serving):

- Calories 284
- Fat 23.4 g
- Carbohydrates 8.9 g
- Sugar 2.2 g
- Protein 12.5 g
- Cholesterol 57 mg

Made in the USA
Thornton, CO
05/24/24 20:48:44

dd158202-f539-4f03-b6d9-cdcf673a6899R01